DATE DUE		

STRANGERS DON'T LOOK LIKE THE BIG BAD WOLF

by

Janis Buschman and Debbie Hunley

Foreword by

Linda D. Meyer, Author
of SAFETY ZONE: A Book
Teaching Child Abduction
Prevention Skills.

Illustrations by
Marina Megale

Edited By
Linda D. Meyer and
Carole Lyons

THE CHAS. FRANKLIN PRESS
7821 175th St. S.W., Edmonds, WA 98020

DEDICATION

TO OUR CHILDREN JENNIFER, JESSICA, ALEXA, KENDA

ACKNOWLEDGEMENTS:

We wish to thank Susan McAlexander and J.B. Hunley.

THE CHILDREN'S SAFETY SERIES:

PRIVATE ZONE: A Book Teaching Children Sexual Assault
Prevention Tools by Frances S. Dayee.

SAFETY ZONE: A Book Teaching Child Abduction Prevention
Skills by Linda D. Meyer.

HELP YOURSELF TO SAFETY: A Guide To Avoiding Dangerous
Situations With Strangers and Friends by Kate Hubbard
and Evelyn Berlin.

IT'S NOT YOUR FAULT by Judy Jance.

STRANGERS DON'T LOOK LIKE THE BIG BAD WOLF
by Janis Buschman and Debbie Hunley.

DIAL ZERO FOR HELP: A Story of Parental Kidnapping
by Judy Jance.

ATTENTION: SCHOOLS AND ORGANIZATIONS

Our books are available at quantity discounts
with bulk purchase for educational use.
For information, please write to:
Special Sales Dept., The Chas. Franklin Press,
7821 175th St. S.W., Edmonds, WA 98020.

FOREWORD

Although the beginning of a movement is always hard to pin down, the missing children's movement might be said to have begun in February 1975. At that time Families and Friends of Missing Persons and Violent Crime Victims was founded in Seattle, Washington.

The coming years saw gradual awareness spread through the growth of many more groups: the Society For Young Victims, the National Coalition for Children's Justice, the Dee Scofield Awareness Program, Child Find and many more.

Then in November of 1980 six year old Etan Patz was abducted, and the tragedy became a turning point. Associated Press distributed a release in which Julie and Stanley Patz called for the founding of a national clearing-house for missing children. Agencies from across the U.S. responded, and ACTION, A Confederation To Inform Others Nationally, was founded.

Because of this, the media finally began focusing some attention on the tragedy of our missing children. Articles ran in such magazines as *Family Circle, People, Ladies Home Journal* and in a variety of newspapers nationally. An article which ran in *Reader's Digest* was another landmark. For the first time pictures of missing children were published, and, as a direct result, a missing child was located. There followed the publishing in the media of the pictures of many more lost children.

Then, in July 1981, fate made a mistake if it wanted to keep the whole thing quiet: six year old Adam Walsh was abducted and murdered out of Hollywood, Florida. John and Reve Walsh entered the movement, and the whole thing blew wide open.

The Walshes discovered that the FBI would search for a missing race horse, but would not search for a missing child. They wouldn't track missing children in their computer, but they would track missing cars.

In January 1982 the Adam Walsh Child Resource Center was founded and merged with Child Advocacy which had begun their work in 1973. The Walshes were a vital, explosive force in the missing children's movement, and, after pounding on innumerable doors and giving innumerable talks, John's efforts lead to the Missing Children's Act which was signed into law in October 1982. This piece of legislation allowed (though did not mandate) the FBI to accept information on missing children from parents when the local police do not provide it.

John Walsh's first three years were frustrating as he continued to try to get people to listen, to hear, to believe that the abduction and sexual exploitation of our children is a real thing, and not some figment of an angry and grieving father's overactive imagination. Only now have people finally begun to listen. And to act.

Pictures of missing children can now be found on posters in department stores, on milk cartons, pizza boxes and grocery bags, and even plastered across the side of a convoy of trucks. People are finally believing.

When Safety Zone came out in 1984 after I view the dramatic story of ADAM, there were no other books available. Now, thankfully, there are many, and each contributes in its way to making our children safer from abduction and exploitation. STRANGERS DON'T LOOK LIKE THE BIG BAD WOLF is another fine example. Whereas Safety Zone taught abduction prevention to elementary school age children, STRANGERS was designed especially for toddlers and pre-schoolers. Your children will learn vital information while enjoying the story of Molly.

The proliferation of books in the movement is welcome, but one other thing is critical, and that is a mandatory change of adult attitudes. We can no longer teach our children that ALL big people are nice. They are NOT! WHEN WE TEACH OUR CHILDREN TO ALWAYS RESPECT AND OBEY ADULTS, WE ARE INADVERTENTLY SETTING THEM UP FOR A POTENTIAL ABDUCTION OR MOLESTATION. We make our children vulnerable with this attitude.

We must watch our words. To leave our children at home or at school saying, "Now you be sure to mind the babysitter (or teacher)" leaves our children vulnerable. Instead we must teach them as they grow older that their bodies are private and to recognize potentially dangerous situations. There is much we must change about the way we teach our young ones.

Children are our treasures. We would do well to begin to think of ourselves as but guardians. Children are not our possessions. They belong to God.

Linda D. Meyer, author
SAFETY ZONE: A Book
Teaching Abduction
Prevention Skills

ADULT'S PAGE

To the very young child, the word stranger holds no special meaning. To these children, all faces are friendly. Then how do we make them aware of the dangers of child abduction? This is the reason we have written STRANGERS DON'T LOOK LIKE THE BIG BAD WOLF! In educating our pre-schoolers, it is not our goal to frighten them or to ask them to make value judgments. Rather, by taking every-day situations and presenting them in story form, our young children can learn the importance of STAYING NEAR A SAFE PERSON, e.g. Babysitter, Grandparents.

We would like to recommend that parents use this picture book over and over with their children. This can be taken a step further by making up your own stories to fit your child's activities. As a parent, familiarize yourself with the lures most commonly used in child abduction (see appendix). Realize that YOU are your pre-school child's only real defense. Left alone, there is no guarantee of safety.

Almost daily, the American public is made more and more aware of the rise in child abduction. Now and then it is with you that we hear the report of a missing child's being reunited with his parents. However, it is far more often that we hear the stories told by grieving parents whose young-sters have been missing for months or years.

Much is being done today to help locate missing children. Efforts are being made to educate parents and children concerning child abduction, its most common lures, and how to avoid them. Yet, statistics still remain too high. Child Find reports that up to 500,000 children are abducted each year by a non-custodial parent and 2,000 to 6,000 by strangers.

Our children are our greatest assets, our most precious treasures. They are worth any time and effort we can give to protect them from such a horrendous crime as child abduction.

STRANGERS DON'T
LOOK LIKE
THE BIG BAD WOLF

Most people in the world
are nice and friendly.

Some nice and friendly
people are strangers.

Strangers don't look like monsters!

Strangers don't look like
the big bad wolf!

Strangers look just like everybody else!
HOORAY FOR MOLLY because she's
learning all about strangers.

1

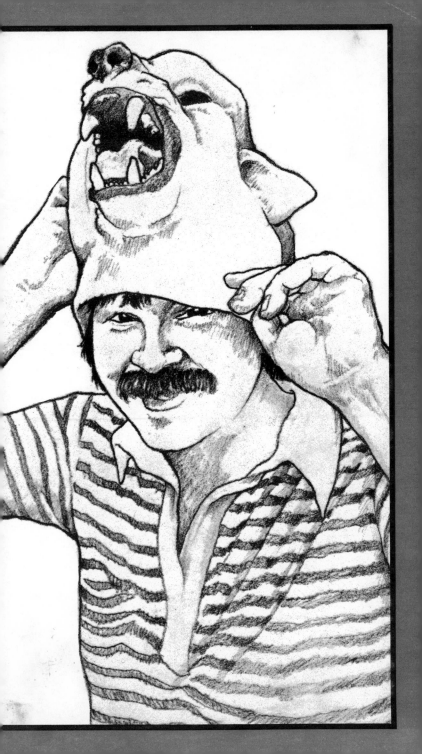

It was Monday and Molly was playing
at her preschool while her Mommy
and Daddy went to work.

That afternoon, a **nice** lady came
to get Molly. This lady did not
look like a monster, she did not
look like a big bad wolf,
but she WAS a stranger!
Can you guess what Molly did?

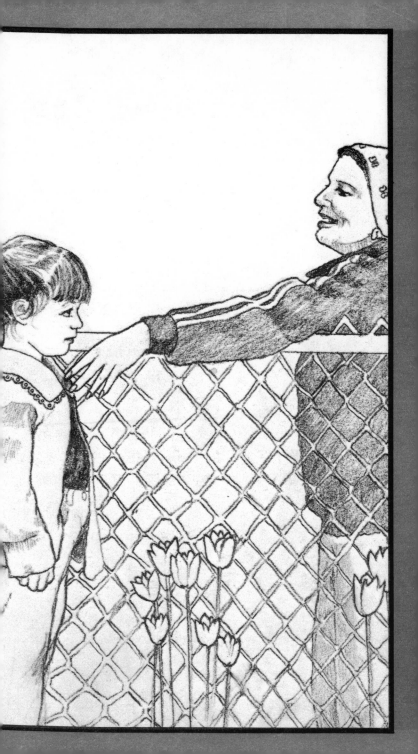

Molly ran as fast as she could to her teacher and yelled, "NO! I'll wait here with my teacher!"

HOORAY FOR MOLLY!
She knows her teacher would **never** want her to leave the preschool with a stranger.

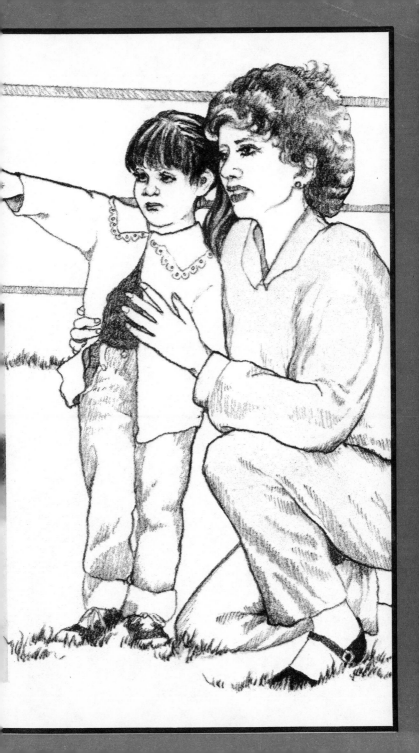

On Tuesday, Molly was outside playing when a nice man drove up in a car. He asked Molly for directions to the park and then said, "You can have this puppy if you will show me the way." Can you guess what Molly did?

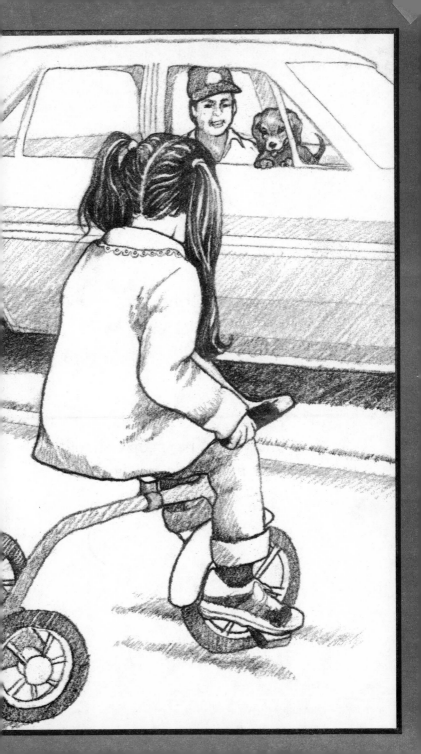

Molly jumped off her tricycle and
ran as fast as she could to get
her Mommy.

HOORAY FOR MOLLY!
She knows that big people should
ask other big people for directions,
NOT little children.

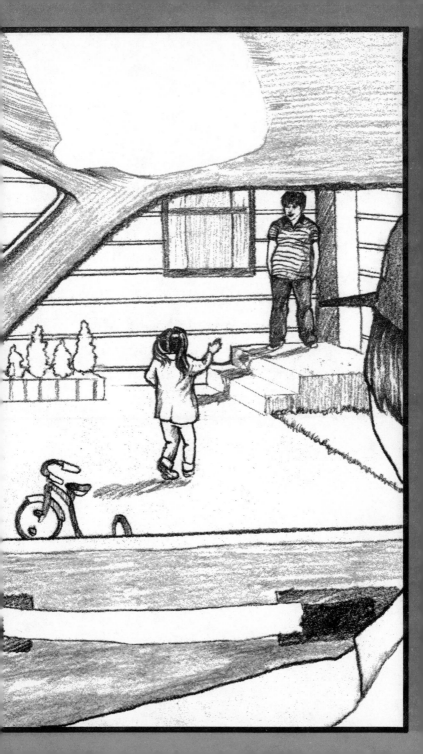

On Wednesday, Molly and Mike were playing in Grandmother's backyard. Mike said, "Molly! Look! There's the trash truck! Let's go out to the alley and watch!"
Can you guess what Molly did?

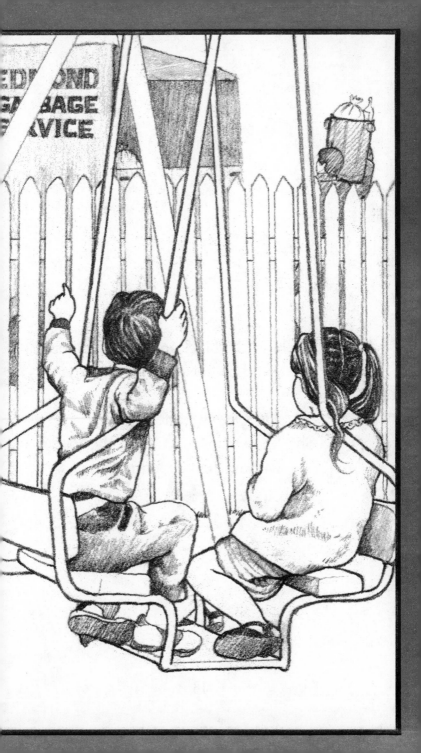

Molly said, "No!" and ran as fast as she could to get her Grandmother.

HOORAY FOR MOLLY!
She knows never to leave the yard without her Grandmother.

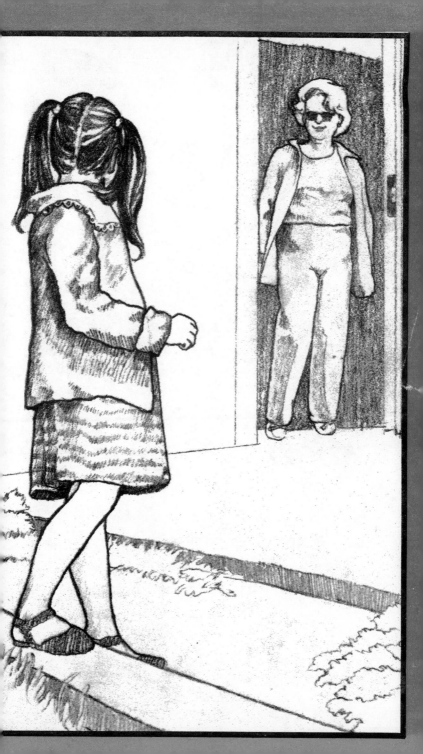

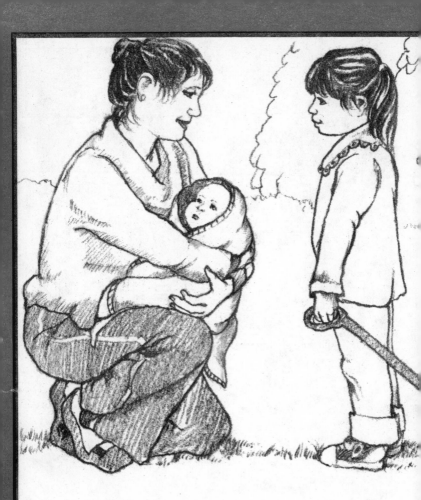

On Thursday, Molly was outside
giving her baby doll a ride
in the red wagon.
"Hello, Mrs. Miller. See my new
baby doll?"

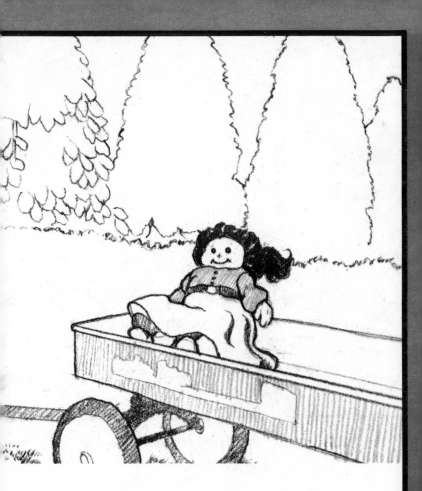

"What a pretty baby," said Mrs.
Miller. "Why don't you
come inside my house and help me
feed **my** new baby?"
Can you guess what Molly did?

Molly ran as fast as she could and
asked her Mommy if she could go
see Mrs. Miller's baby.

HOORAY FOR MOLLY! She
knows to always ask her Mommy
first before she goes anywhere with
a good friend.

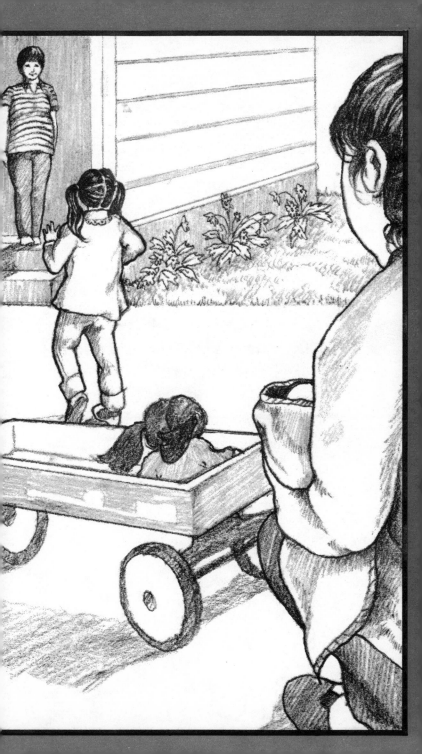

Friday was a special day.
Molly and her Daddy were going
to the fair.

"This is fun!" said Molly. "I want
to ride the merry-go-round!"
Can you guess what Molly did?

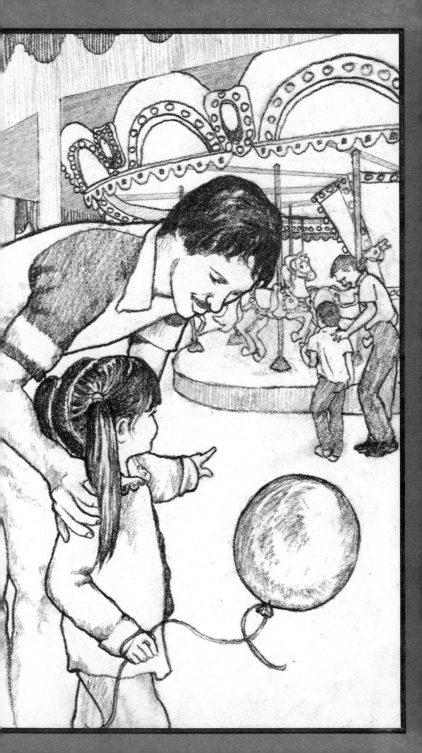

Molly reached up, grabbed her
Daddy's hand and pulled him as
fast as she could to
the merry-go-round.

HOORAY FOR MOLLY!
She remembered to stay
with her Daddy
when she's in a crowded place.

Crowded places are full of strangers
and Molly knows . . . .

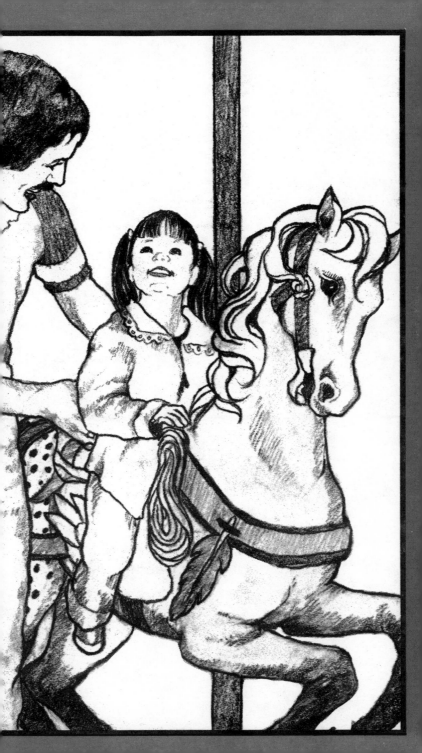

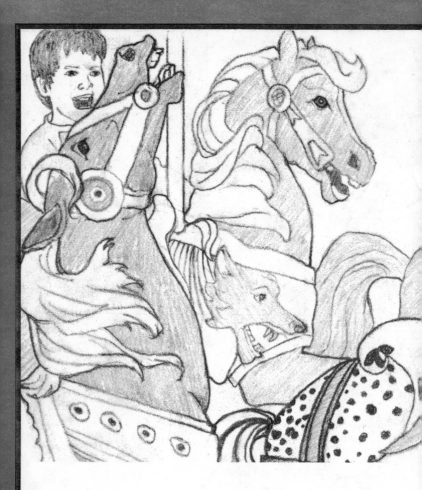

Strangers don't look like monsters!
Strangers don't look like the big
bad wolf! Strangers look just like

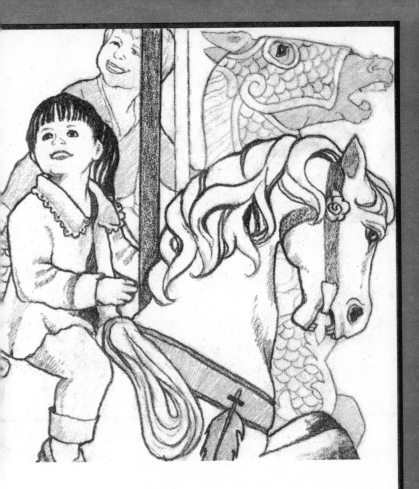

everybody else!
HIP HIP HOORAY FOR MOLLY!!!

The End

GUIDELINES FOR PARENTS

A. The very young child should always be in clear view and supervised by an adult, especially when he is at a park, grocery store, fair, or any type of public place.

B. Remember that carnivals, fairs, public restrooms, and malls are the most common places where abductions occur.

C. Be sure you know where your child is and when to expect him home.

D. Always go with your child to the restroom when in a public place.

E. Never leave your child alone in a car.

F. Consider placing locks on any gates which would easily be opened by your young child.

G. Be sure your child does not wear any clothing item which has his name printed, monogrammed, or painted on, since this could be used to convince the child that this stranger knows him.

H. Be sure your child's care facility will not allow him to leave with anyone other than you, without your prior permission.

I. Consider obtaining a passport for your child. In the event that your child is abducted, it will help prevent him from being taken out of the U.S. the passport office should be notified and help in finding missing children.

J. Keep records on your child which include their fingerprints, blood type, lock of hair, recent picture, and dental records.

K. Be sure your child's name and picture do not appear together in the newspaper.

L. Write on the tags of your child's clothing, his name, address, area code and telephone number.

M. If your child disappears, call the police. If he is not found promptly, make sure the police file a missing persons report with the F.B.I. If they fail to do this, be sure you do it yourself.

N. Teach your child to come tell you when something bad happens to him.

O. When in public places, give your child specific instructions on where to meet you in case of separation, such as customer service, cash register, fountain, etc.

GUIDELINES FOR YOUNG CHILDREN

Below are some suggestions you can start teaching your young child. Some of these suggestions may be too difficult for him to learn immediately, depending on his age and ability. However, eventually he will be able to learn and comprehend all of these suggestions, at which time he will be a much safer and better informed child.

Your child should learn:

a. his first and last name and his parents' first and last names.

b. his street address, city, state, area code, and phone number.

c. he is safer when in a group. Explain the "Buddy System."

d. to kick and scream if anyone ever grabs his arms or tries to pick him up and carry him away.

e. what to do if he ever has to answer the phone or door.

f. he has your permission to say "NO" to adults.

g. never to leave with anyone, including your divorced spouse or even a friend, without your permission.

h. never to leave his own yard without your permission.

i. to stay close to you when in a crowded place.

j. a secret code word to be used as a signal if you send an unfamiliar adult to pick him up.

k. the physical boundaries to stay within while playing in unfenced areas.

l. to dial "O" in case of an emergency.

WHAT IF . . .

For most children, the ability to generalize does not develop until they reach their pre-teen years. Without this ability, children cannot apply the lessons learned from one situation to another similar one. Therefore, it is important to discuss with children how to respond in a responsible manner to a wide variety of potentially dangerous situations. You can use the following situations and make up some of your own. Discuss the best response. Unless otherwise noted the correct response is to always check with a responsible adult, i.e. Mommy or Daddy. Make it into a game.

WHAT WOULD YOU DO IF .....

You are playing ball at a friend's house while Mommy visits. Your ball accidentally goes through a hole in the fence. Your friend says "Let's go get it."

You are playing with a puppy outside. It gets out of the yard.

You are in a cart in the grocery store. A nice lady comes up and asks you your name.

Your Daddy takes you to a movie. It is very crowded. You see the popcorn machine and want some popcorn.

You're at the zoo. You want to go look at the tigers.

A teenager asks you to go to the restroom with him/her.

You're at a playground swinging while your baby-sitter sits on a bench visiting and a man comes and picks you up off the swing. (Scream, yell, bite, kick)

You're at the Library and you want a drink of water.

You're at pre-school and a nice man comes and says, "Your Daddy asked me to come and get you."

A man flashes a badge and says he has to take you to the police station. (Professional lurers can purchase badges through the mail, so the child should always check with another adult).

QUESTIONS

After reading Strangers with your children, it might be useful to ascertain their understanding of the material by asking some questions. Questions will serve an additional purpose: You should make it clear that what happened to Molly is not just a story, but could happen to them. Take it out of the hypothetical and put it into the concrete. Examples are:

1) Did Molly do the right thing?

2) Who are the safe people that Molly ran to?

3) Who are the safe people you could run to?

4) Molly's a girl. Could it happen to boys too?

ADDITIONAL RESOURCES

The following resources teach basic personal safety techniques to children and adults. They may cover abduction as well as sexual assault prevention.

BOOKS

The Children's Safety Series:

PRIVATE ZONE: A Book Teaching Children Sexual Assault Prevention Skills by Frances S. Dayee, Warner Books, 1982.

SAFETY ZONE: A Book Teaching Child Abduction Prevention Skills by Linda D. Meyer, Warner Books, 1985.

HELP YOURSELF TO SAFETY by Kate Hubbard and Evelyn Berlin, 1985, The Chas. Franklin Press, 7821 175th St. S.W., Edmonds, WA 98020, $3.50.

IT'S NOT YOUR FAULT by Judy Jance, 1985, The Chas. Franklin Press, 7821 175th St. S.W., Edmonds, WA 98020, $3.50.

STRANGERS DON'T LOOK LIKE THE BIG BAD WOLF by Janis Buschman and Debbie Hunley, 1985, The Chas. Franklin Press, 7821 175th St. S.W., Edmonds, WA 98020, $3.50.

DIAL ZERO FOR HELP by Judith Jance, 1985, The Chas. Franklin Press, 7821 175th St. S.W., Edmonds, WA 98020, $3.50.

OTHER BOOKS:

IT'S MY BODY: A Book To Teach Young Children How To Resist Uncomfortable Touch by Lory Freeman, 1984, Parenting Press, 7750 31st Ave. N.E., Seattle, WA 98115, $3.00.

PROTECT YOUR CHILD FROM SEXUAL ABUSE by Janie Hart-Rossi, 1984, Parenting Press, 7750 31st Ave. N.E., Seattle, WA 98115, $5.00.

YOUR CHILD SHOULD KNOW by Flora Colao and Tamar Hosansky, The Bobbs-Merrill Company, 1984.

AUDIO-VISUAL MATERIAL:

BOYS BEWARE, AIMS Media, 6901 Woodley Ave., Van Nuys, CA 91406.

GIRLS BEWARE, AIMS Media, 6901 Woodley Ave., Van Nuys, CA 91406.

SAFETY WITH STRANGERS, Adam Walsh Child Resource Center, 1876 N. University Drive, Suite 306, Fort Lauderdale, FL 33322.

STRONG KIDS SAFE KIDS, Henry Winkler; Paramont.

ORGANIZATIONS:

Adam Walsh Child Resource Center
1876 N. University Drive, #306
Ft. Lauderdale, FL 33322
(305) 475-4847

Child Find
P.O. Box 277
New Paltz, NY 12561
(800) 431-5005

Child Find of British Columbia
P.O. Box 34008
Station D
Vancouver, B.C. V6S 4W8

Child Find of Canada
Box G145, Station G
Calgary, Alberta T3B 3B7

Dee Scofoeld Awareness Program, Inc.
4418 Bay Court Ave.
Tampa, FL 33611
(813) 839-5025

National Center for Missing and Exploited Children
1835 K Street N.W., #700
Washington, D.C. 20006
(202) 634-9821

Families and Friends of Missing Persons and
    Violent Crime Victims
Jane Addams Building
11051 34th Ave. N.E.
Seattle, WA 98125
(206) 362-1081

WORKSHOPS/CURRICULUM

S.A.F.E.
541 Avenue of the Americas
New York, NY 10011
(212) 242-4874

T.I.P.S.
Jefferson Bldg.
Fourth Street N.W.
Charlottesville, VA 22901

Committee For Children
P.O. Box 51049
Seattle, WA 98115
(206) 522-5834

Survival Skills For Children
18509 85th Ave. West
Edmonds, WA 98020
(206) 778-9368